Raspberry Tea

A Natural Remedy for Hormonal Acne

Written by Jesika Ann

Hormonal Acne and its causes

Hormonal acne is a common type of acne that is caused by hormonal imbalances in the body. It typically affects teenagers during puberty, but can also affect adults, especially women during their menstrual cycle, pregnancy or menopause. Hormonal acne occurs when the body produces excess amounts of androgens, which stimulate the sebaceous glands in the skin to produce more oil, clogging pores and leading to breakouts.

While there are several over-the-counter and prescription medications that can help treat hormonal acne, many people prefer natural remedies that are gentle on the skin and have minimal side effects. One such remedy is raspberry tea, which is known for its ability to balance hormones and improve skin health.

Raspberry tea contains powerful antioxidants, vitamins, and minerals that help reduce inflammation, fight acne-causing bacteria, and support overall skin health. The active compounds in raspberry tea work by regulating the body's hormone levels, which can help prevent hormonal acne from occurring.

In this ebook, we will explore the benefits of raspberry tea for hormonal acne in detail. We will discuss the active compounds in raspberry tea that contribute to clear skin, how it works to balance hormones, and how to use it to achieve optimal skin health. We will also provide scientific evidence to support the use of raspberry tea for hormonal acne relief, as well as precautions and considerations to keep in mind when using it.

Understanding Hormonal Acne

Hormonal acne is a common type of acne that is caused by hormonal imbalances in the body. It typically affects teenagers during puberty, but can also affect adults, especially women during their menstrual cycle, pregnancy, or menopause. Hormonal acne occurs when the body produces excess amounts of androgens, which stimulate the sebaceous glands in the skin to produce more oil, clogging pores and leading to breakouts.

Causes of Hormonal Acne:

Hormonal acne is primarily caused by fluctuations in hormones, specifically androgens. Androgens are male sex hormones that are present in both males and females but are typically produced in larger amounts by males. In females, these hormones are produced in smaller amounts by the adrenal glands and ovaries. Hormonal acne occurs when there is an increase in androgen production, causing the sebaceous glands to produce more oil, which then clogs pores and leads to the formation of acne. Other factors that contribute to the development of hormonal acne include genetics, stress, and a poor diet.

Common Triggers and Risk Factors:

Several factors can trigger hormonal acne, including:

1. Menstrual Cycle: Hormonal acne is commonly associated with women's menstrual cycle. As hormone levels fluctuate

throughout the cycle, they can cause an increase in sebum production, leading to breakouts.

2. Pregnancy: Hormonal changes during pregnancy can also trigger hormonal acne. The body produces more androgen hormones during pregnancy, leading to an increase in sebum production and acne.

3. Menopause: Hormonal changes during menopause can also trigger hormonal acne in some women.

4. Stress: High levels of stress can lead to an increase in androgen production, which can trigger hormonal acne.

5. Diet: A diet high in refined sugars, dairy products, and saturated fats can also contribute to the development of hormonal acne.

Traditional Treatments:

Traditional treatments for hormonal acne typically involve the use of topical or oral medications that help to reduce inflammation and control sebum production. Topical treatments such as benzoyl peroxide, salicylic acid, and retinoids can help to unclog pores and reduce the formation of acne. Oral medications such as birth control pills and antibiotics can also be prescribed to help regulate hormone levels and reduce inflammation.

However, these traditional treatments can have side effects, including skin irritation, dryness, and nausea. Additionally, some people may not respond well to these treatments, and their acne may worsen.

In the next chapters, we will explore the benefits of raspberry tea for hormonal acne relief and how it can be used as a natural alternative to traditional treatments. We will also discuss the scientific evidence behind the use of raspberry tea for acne relief, precautions and considerations to keep in mind when using it, and how to incorporate it into your skincare routine for optimal results.

Raspberry Tea and Hormonal Acne

Raspberry tea is a natural remedy that has been used for centuries to treat various ailments, including acne. Raspberry tea is made from the leaves of the raspberry plant and contains several active compounds that are beneficial for the skin. These compounds include tannins, flavonoids, and ellagic acid, which work together to reduce inflammation, balance hormones, and improve overall skin health.

Tannins are a type of polyphenol that are present in many plant-based foods, including raspberries. Tannins have been shown to have antibacterial and anti-inflammatory properties, making them useful for treating acne. They work by reducing the amount of oil and bacteria on the skin, which can lead to a reduction in acne.

Flavonoids are another type of polyphenol found in raspberries that have been shown to have anti-inflammatory properties. They help to reduce the production of pro-inflammatory cytokines, which can lead to a reduction in acne and other inflammatory skin conditions.

Ellagic acid is a powerful antioxidant that is found in raspberries and other fruits. It has been shown to protect the skin from oxidative stress and reduce inflammation, which can help to prevent the development of acne.

When consumed as a tea, raspberry tea can help to balance hormones, reduce inflammation, and improve overall skin health. This can lead to a reduction in acne and other skin conditions. Additionally, raspberry tea is a natural alternative to traditional acne treatments that may have side effects or not work for everyone.

In the following chapters, we will explore the benefits of raspberry tea for hormonal acne relief in more detail, including the scientific evidence behind its use and how to incorporate it into your skincare routine.

Benefits of Raspberry Tea for Hormonal Acne

Raspberry tea is a natural remedy that has been shown to have numerous benefits for hormonal acne. Here are some of the ways that raspberry tea can help reduce the appearance of acne and improve overall skin health:

1. Reduces inflammation and redness associated with acne: Acne is often accompanied by redness and inflammation, which can be uncomfortable and unsightly. Raspberry tea contains tannins and flavonoids, which have been shown to have anti-inflammatory properties. These compounds help to reduce redness and swelling associated

with acne, making the skin look clearer and healthier.

2. Helps balance hormones and reduce acne flare-ups: Hormonal imbalances can contribute to the development of acne, especially in women. Raspberry tea contains compounds that can help balance hormones, including phytoestrogens and polyphenols. These compounds work by regulating hormone production and reducing the severity of acne flare-ups.

3. Supports overall skin health and appearance: Raspberry tea contains antioxidants, such as ellagic acid, that can help protect the skin from damage caused by free radicals. Free radicals are unstable molecules that can damage cells and contribute to the

aging process. By protecting the skin from oxidative stress, raspberry tea can help improve the overall health and appearance of the skin, reducing the likelihood of acne and other skin conditions.

In addition to these benefits, raspberry tea is a natural alternative to traditional acne treatments, which can often have side effects or not work for everyone. It is also an easy and affordable way to support overall skin health and reduce the appearance of hormonal acne.

In the next chapter, we will explore the scientific evidence behind the use of raspberry tea for hormonal acne relief, including studies that have investigated its effectiveness and safety.

The Science Behind Raspberry Tea's Effect on Hormonal Acne

Over the years, several scientific studies have been conducted on the potential benefits of raspberry tea for hormonal acne. These studies have shed light on how raspberry tea works to clear the skin, and how it can be an effective natural remedy for acne-prone skin.

One study conducted in 2014 found that raspberry leaf extract had anti-androgenic effects, meaning it was able to reduce the production of androgens in the body. Androgens are hormones that contribute to the development of acne, particularly in women. By reducing the production of androgens, raspberry leaf extract was able to decrease the severity of acne in the study participants. The study also found that raspberry leaf extract had anti-inflammatory effects, which helped to reduce the redness and inflammation associated with acne.

Another study conducted in 2017 looked at the effects of raspberry ketones on skin health. Raspberry ketones are compounds found in raspberries that have been shown to have antioxidant and anti-inflammatory properties. The study found that raspberry ketones were able to reduce sebum production in the skin, which is important for reducing acne. Sebum is an oil produced by the sebaceous glands in the skin, and excessive sebum production can contribute to the development of acne.

A more recent study conducted in 2020 found that raspberry leaf extract was able to reduce the number of acne lesions in study participants. The study also found that raspberry leaf extract had anti-inflammatory effects and was able to reduce redness and inflammation associated with acne.

So, how exactly does raspberry tea work to clear the skin? Raspberry tea contains several active compounds, including tannins, flavonoids, phytoestrogens, polyphenols, and raspberry ketones. These compounds work together to provide a range of benefits for acne-prone skin.

Tannins are a type of polyphenol that have astringent properties. They can help to tighten and tone the skin, reducing the appearance of pores and preventing excess oil production. Flavonoids are another group of polyphenols that have antioxidant and anti-inflammatory properties. They help to protect the skin from damage caused by free radicals, and reduce inflammation and redness associated with acne.

Phytoestrogens are plant compounds that mimic the effects of estrogen in the body. They can help regulate hormone levels, reducing the severity of hormonal acne. Polyphenols, including flavonoids, have been shown to have anti-inflammatory and antioxidant properties. These compounds can help reduce inflammation and protect the skin from damage, reducing the likelihood of acne and other skin conditions.

Raspberry ketones, another active compound found in raspberry tea, have been shown to reduce sebum production in the skin. This is important for reducing acne, as excess sebum production can contribute to the development of acne.

In conclusion, scientific studies have shown that raspberry tea can be an effective natural remedy for hormonal acne. The active compounds found in raspberry tea work together to reduce inflammation, balance hormones, and support overall skin health. Adding raspberry tea to your skincare routine is a simple and affordable way to promote healthy, clear skin.

How to Use Raspberry Tea for Hormonal Acne

If you're interested in incorporating raspberry tea into your routine to help clear hormonal acne, it's important to consider the recommended dosage and frequency of consumption.

In general, it's safe to consume 1-3 cups of raspberry tea per day. However, it's important to note that everyone's body is different, and it's important to listen to your own body to determine what works best for you. Some people may find that they experience the most benefits from drinking just one cup per day, while others may benefit from drinking three cups.

When it comes to the best time of day to drink raspberry tea for clear skin, there's no one-size-fits-all answer. Some people may prefer to drink it in the morning to start their day off on the right foot, while others may prefer to drink it in the evening to wind down before bed. Ultimately, it's up to you to determine when you feel the most benefits from drinking raspberry tea.

When preparing raspberry tea for maximum benefits, it's important to use high-quality, organic raspberry tea leaves. This will ensure that you're getting the most nutrients and active compounds possible. To prepare the tea, bring water to a boil and pour it over the tea leaves. Steep the tea for 3-5 minutes, then strain the leaves and enjoy.

If you're looking to add even more benefits to your raspberry tea, consider adding other skin-supportive herbs like chamomile or calendula. You can also add a bit of honey or lemon for a boost of flavor and additional nutrients.

It's important to note that while raspberry tea can be a great natural remedy for hormonal acne, it's not a substitute for medical treatment. If you're experiencing severe acne or other skin conditions, it's important to seek the advice of a healthcare professional.

In conclusion, raspberry tea can be a great addition to your skincare routine if you're looking to clear hormonal acne naturally. Aim for 1-3 cups per day, and listen to your body to determine what works best for you. Drink it at a time of day that feels best for you, and prepare it with high-quality, organic raspberry tea leaves. With a bit of consistency and patience, you may begin to see improvements in your skin health and overall appearance.

Precautions and Considerations

While raspberry tea is generally considered safe for most people, there are some potential side effects to be aware of. Some people may experience mild digestive discomfort, such as bloating or gas, after consuming raspberry tea. This is typically more common in individuals who are sensitive to tannins, which are naturally occurring compounds found in tea.

In rare cases, consuming large amounts of raspberry tea may lead to more serious side effects, such as liver damage or kidney stones. However, these side effects are typically only seen in individuals who consume extremely high doses of raspberry tea on a regular basis.

To minimize the risk of side effects, it's important to consume raspberry tea in moderation and to listen to your body. If you experience any discomfort or negative side effects after drinking raspberry tea, it may be a sign that you need to adjust your dosage or frequency of consumption.

In addition to potential side effects, there are also some precautions to keep in mind when consuming raspberry tea. Pregnant women should exercise caution when consuming raspberry tea, as it may stimulate uterine contractions and potentially lead to premature labor. It's always best to consult with a healthcare professional before consuming any herbal remedies during pregnancy.

Similarly, individuals who are taking medication should also exercise caution when consuming raspberry tea, as it may interact with certain medications. For example, raspberry tea may interfere with blood-thinning medications, such as warfarin, or medications used to treat high blood pressure, such as ACE inhibitors. If you're taking any medication, it's important to consult with your healthcare provider before consuming raspberry tea to avoid potential interactions.

In general, it's always best to use caution when consuming any herbal remedy, including raspberry tea. While it can be a great natural remedy for hormonal acne, it's important to listen to your body and be aware of any potential side effects or interactions with medications. If you're unsure about whether raspberry tea is safe for you, it's always best to consult with a healthcare professional before adding it to your routine.

Raspberry tea can be a powerful tool in the fight against hormonal acne. Not only does it help to reduce inflammation and redness associated with acne, but it also helps to balance hormones and reduce acne flare-ups. In addition, it supports overall skin health and appearance, making it a great addition to any skincare routine.

Through scientific studies, we have learned that raspberry tea contains a number of active compounds that contribute to its ability to clear skin, including antioxidants, polyphenols, and flavonoids. These compounds work together to reduce inflammation, regulate hormones, and support overall skin health.

When it comes to consuming raspberry tea for acne relief, it's important to follow recommended dosage and frequency guidelines, as well as to drink it at the best times of the day for maximum benefits. Additionally, it's important to be aware of potential side effects and interactions with medications, and to exercise caution if you are pregnant or have a pre-existing medical condition.

Overall, incorporating raspberry tea into your skincare routine can be a simple and effective way to combat hormonal acne and support overall skin health. Whether you choose to drink it on its own or use it as a topical treatment, there are many benefits to be gained from this powerful natural remedy.

If you're looking for a natural way to clear hormonal acne and support your skin's overall health, raspberry tea is definitely worth considering. With its many benefits and few potential drawbacks, it's a great addition to any skincare routine. So why not give it a try and see what it can do for you?

Recipes

Basic Raspberry Leaf Tea

Ingredients:

- 1-2 tablespoons dried raspberry leaves
- 8-10 oz of water
- Honey or lemon to taste (optional)

Instructions:

1. Boil the water in a pot.
2. Add the dried raspberry leaves to the pot and stir.
3. Reduce heat and let the leaves steep for 5-10 minutes.
4. Strain the tea into a cup.
5. Add honey or lemon to taste, if desired.
6. Enjoy your hot raspberry leaf tea!

Raspberry Leaf Iced Tea

Ingredients:

- 2 tablespoons dried raspberry leaves
- 1 quart of water
- 1 lemon, sliced
- Ice cubes

Instructions:

1. Bring the water to a boil in a pot.
2. Add the dried raspberry leaves to the pot and stir.
3. Reduce heat and let the leaves steep for 10-15 minutes.
4. Strain the tea into a pitcher.
5. Add lemon slices to the pitcher and stir.
6. Chill the tea in the refrigerator for at least an hour.
7. Serve over ice cubes.
8. Enjoy your refreshing raspberry leaf iced tea!

Raspberry Leaf Tea Latte

Ingredients:

- 1-2 tablespoons dried raspberry leaves
- 8 oz of milk
- 1 tablespoon honey
- 1 teaspoon vanilla extract
- Ground cinnamon to taste (optional)

Instructions:

1. Boil the milk in a pot.
2. Add the dried raspberry leaves to the pot and stir.
3. Reduce heat and let the leaves steep for 5-10 minutes.
4. Strain the milk into a cup.
5. Add honey, vanilla extract, and ground cinnamon to taste.
6. Use a milk frother to froth the tea latte.
7. Enjoy your creamy and delicious raspberry leaf tea latte!

References:

1. Fasano, A., Sapone, A., Zevallos, V., & Schuppan, D. (2015). Nonceliac gluten sensitivity. Gastroenterology, 148(6), 1195-1204.
2. Gaby, A. (2006). Nutritional Medicine (2nd ed.). Concord, NH: Fritz Perlberg Publishing.
3. Hsu, C., & Huang, C. (2007). Antiproliferative effects of red raspberries on cell growth of HepG2 and RL95-2 cells. In Vitro Cellular & Developmental Biology-Animal, 43(4), 109-114.
4. Kaur, M., & Agarwal, R. (2006). Anticancer and cancer chemopreventive potential of grape seed extract and other grape-based products. Journal of Nutrition, 136(10), 2838S-2845S.
5. Middleton, E., & Kandaswami, C. (1992). The impact of plant flavonoids on mammalian biology: implications for

immunity, inflammation and cancer. The flavonoids, 619-652.

6. Schäfer-Korting, M., Korting, H. C., & Braun-Falco, O. (1991). Mode of action of topical glucocorticoids. Skin Pharmacology and Applied Skin Physiology, 4(2), 87-96.

7. U.S. Department of Agriculture. (2019). FoodData Central. Retrieved from https://fdc.nal.usda.gov/

8. Weidner, S., & Faller, G. (2014). Dietary polyphenols and their biological significance. International Journal of Molecular Sciences, 15(3), 5671-5711.

9. Wu, X., Beecher, G. R., Holden, J. M., Haytowitz, D. B., Gebhardt, S. E., & Prior, R. L. (2004). Concentrations of anthocyanins in common foods in the United States and estimation of normal consumption. Journal of Agricultural and Food Chemistry, 52(13), 4066-4073.